The New Mediterranean

Recipe Book

Fit and Healthy Everyday Recipes To Improve Your Health and Live Well

Alison Russell

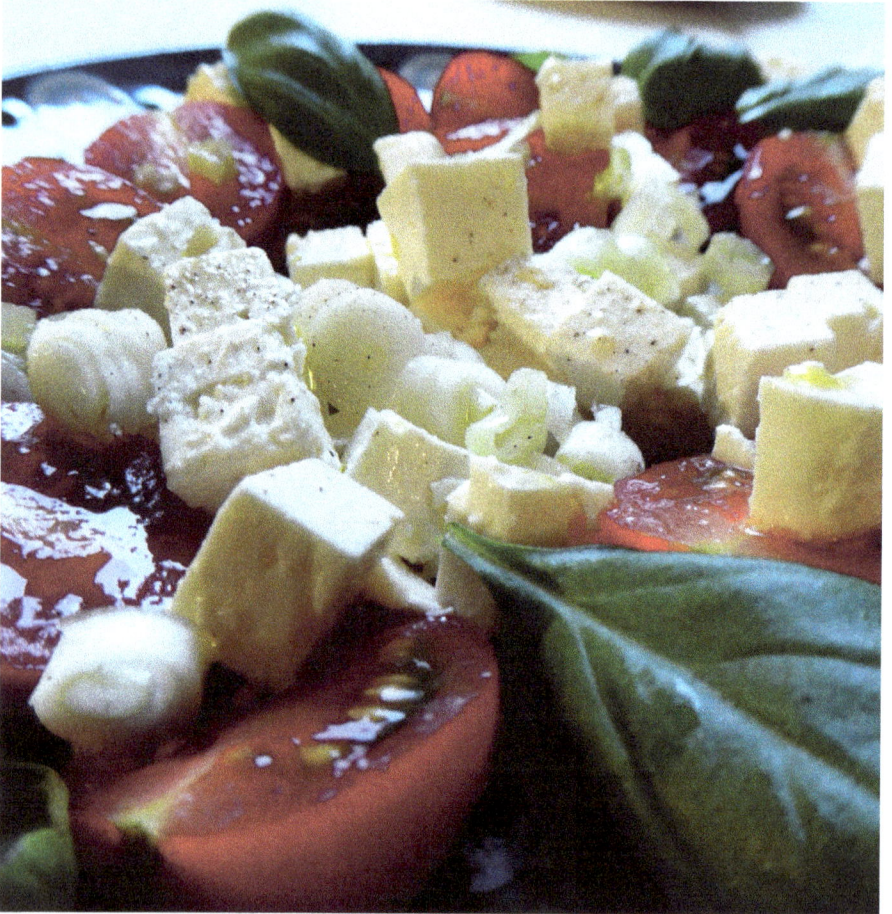

Table of contents

Breakfast

Classic Shakshouka-Style Mediterranean Breakfast

Preparation Time: 10 minutes

Cooking Time: 20 minutes

Servings: 2

Ingredients:

- Parsley, one tablespoon, chopped finely
- Eggs, four
- Olive oil, two tablespoons
- Chili sauce any variety, one teaspoon
- Black pepper, one teaspoon
- Tomatoes, two cups, chopped
- Salt, one-half of one teaspoon
- Garlic, two cloves, chopped finely
- Onion, one large yellow, shredded thinly
- Red bell peppers, two, shredded thinly

Directions:

1. Cook the garlic, peppers, and onions for five minutes in the olive oil.
2. Mix in the chili sauce and the tomatoes; cook for five more minutes.
3. Sprinkle in the pepper and salt.

11

4. Make four round spaces in the mix in the pan, and break the eggs gently into the spaces.
5. Cook for five minutes until the eggs are set.

Nutrition:

Calories 304; 18.1 grams fat; 623 milligrams sodium; 23.1 grams carbs; 3.8 grams fiber; 1.2 grams sugar; 14.3 grams protein

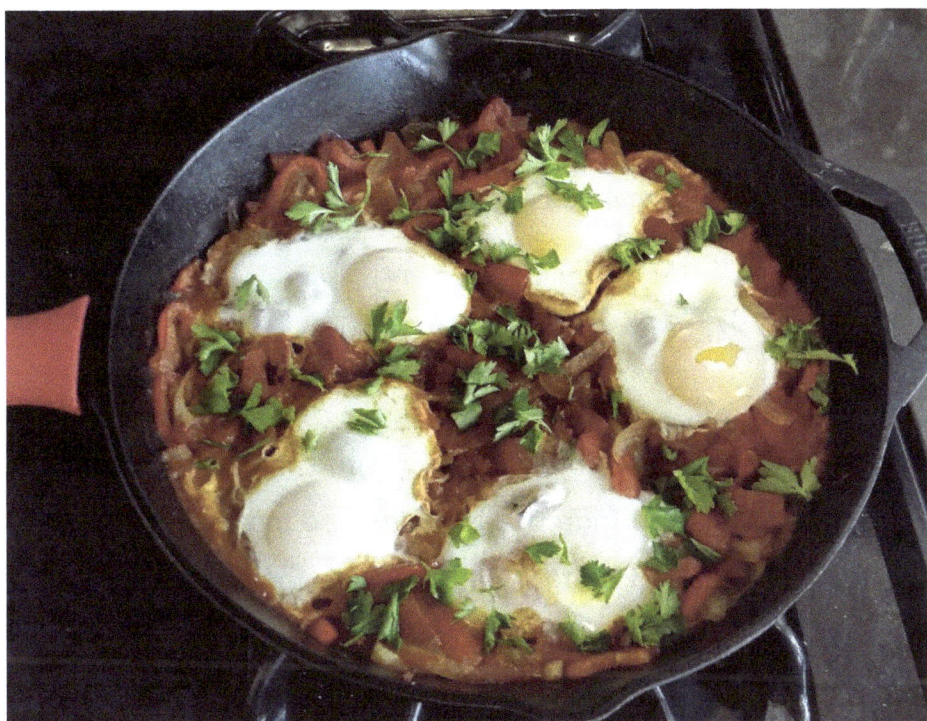

Strawberries Oatmeal

Preparation Time: 5 minutes

Cooking Time: 15 minutes

Servings: 4

Ingredients:

- ½ cup coconut; shredded
- ¼ cup strawberries
- 2 cups coconut milk
- ¼ tsp. vanilla extract
- 2 tsp. stevia

Cooking spray

Directions:

1. Grease the Air Fryer's pan with the cooking spray, add all the Ingredients inside and toss
2. Cook at 365°F for 15 minutes, divide into bowls and serve for breakfast

Nutrition:

Calories: 142

Fat: 7g

Fiber: 2g

Carbs: 3g

Protein: 5g

Chicken Omelet

Preparation Time: 10 minutes

Cooking Time: 16 minutes

Servings: 2

Ingredients:

- 1 teaspoon butter
- 1 small yellow onion, chopped
- ½ jalapeño pepper, seeded and chopped
- 3 eggs
- Salt and ground black pepper, as required
- ¼ cup cooked chicken, shredded

Directions:

1. In a frying pan, melt the butter over medium heat and cook the onion for about 4-5 minutes. Add the jalapeño pepper and cook for about 1 minute.
2. Remove from the heat and set aside to cool slightly. Meanwhile, in a bowl, add the eggs, salt, and black pepper and beat well.
3. Add the onion mixture and chicken and stir to combine. Place the chicken mixture into a small baking pan.
4. Press "Power Button" of Air Fry Oven and turn the dial to select the "Air Fry" mode. Press the Time

button and again turn the dial to set the cooking time to 6 minutes.

5. Now push the Temp button and rotate the dial to set the temperature at 355 degrees F.
6. Press "Start/Pause" button to start.
7. When the unit beeps to show that it is preheated, open the lid.
8. Arrange pan over the "Wire Rack" and insert in the oven.
9. Cut the omelet into 2 portions and serve hot.

Nutrition:

Calories: 153; Total Fat: 9.1 g; Saturated Fat: 3.4 g; Cholesterol: 264 mg; Sodium: 196 mg; Total Carbs: 4 g; Fiber: 0.9 g; Sugar: 2.1 g; Protein: 13.8 g

Zucchini Fritters

Preparation Time: 15 minutes

Cooking Time: 7 minutes

Servings: 2

Ingredients:

- 10½ oz. zucchini, grated and squeezed
- 7 oz. Halloumi cheese
- ¼ cup all-purpose flour
- 2 eggs
- 1 teaspoon fresh dill, minced
- Salt and ground black pepper, as required

Directions:

1. In a large bowl and mix together all the ingredients.
2. Make a small-sized fritter from the mixture.
3. Press "Power Button" of Air Fry Oven and turn the dial to select the "Air Fry" mode.
4. Press the Time button and again turn the dial to set the cooking time to 7 minutes.
5. Now push the Temp button and rotate the dial to set the temperature at 355 degrees F.
6. Press "Start/Pause" button to start.
7. When the unit beeps to show that it is preheated, open the lid.

8. Arrange fritters into grease "Sheet Pan" and insert in the oven.

9. Serve warm.

Nutrition:

Calories: 253; Total Fat: 17.2 g; Saturated Fat: 11 g; Cholesterol: 121 mg; Sodium: 333 mg; Total Carbs: 10 g; Fiber: 1.1 g; Sugar: 2.7 g; Protein: 15.2 g

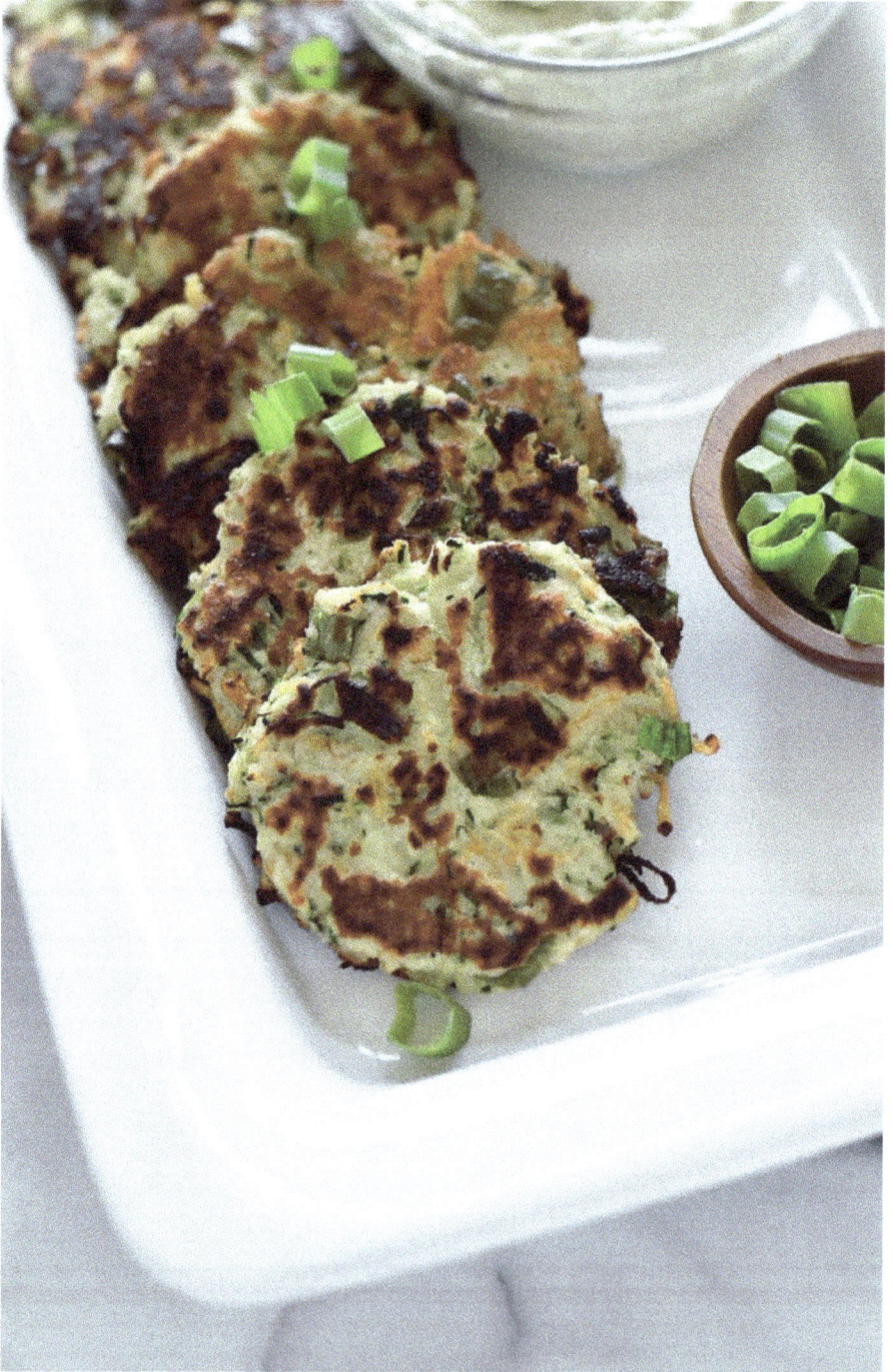

Scrambled Eggs

Preparation Time: 5 minutes

Cooking Time: 20 minutes

Servings: 2

Ingredients:

- 4 large eggs.
- ½ cup shredded sharp Cheddar cheese.
- 2 tbsp. unsalted butter; melted.

Directions:

1. Crack eggs into 2-cup round baking dish and whisk.
2. Place dish into the air fryer basket.
3. Adjust the temperature to 400 Degrees F and set the timer for 10 minutes.
4. After 5 minutes, stir the eggs and add the butter and cheese.
5. Let cook 3 more minutes and stir again.
6. Allow eggs to finish cooking an additional 2 minutes or remove if they are to your desired liking.
7. Use a fork to fluff. Serve warm.

Nutrition:

Calories: 359

Protein: 19.5g

Fiber: 0.0g

Fat: 27.6g

Carbs: 1.1g

Smoked Salmon and Poached Eggs on Toast

Preparation Time: 10 minutes

Cooking Time: 4 minutes

Servings: 4

Ingredients:

- 2 oz avocado smashed
- 2 slices of bread toasted
- Pinch of kosher salt and cracked black pepper
- 1/4 tsp freshly squeezed lemon juice
- 2 eggs see notes, poached
- 3.5 oz smoked salmon
- 1 TBSP. thinly sliced scallions
- Splash of Kikkoman soy sauce optional
- Microgreens are optional

Directions:

1. Take a small bowl and then smash the avocado into it. Then, add the lemon juice and also a pinch of salt into the mixture. Then, mix it well and set aside.

2. After that, poach the eggs and toast the bread for some time. Once the bread is toasted, you will have to spread the avocado on both slices and after that, add the smoked salmon to each slice.

23

3. Thereafter, carefully transfer the poached eggs to the respective toasts. Add a splash of Kikkoman soy sauce and some cracked pepper; then, just garnish with scallions and microgreens.

Nutrition:

Calories: 459

Protein: 31 g

Fat: 22 g

Carbs: 33 g

Honey Almond Ricotta Spread with Peaches

Preparation Time: 5 minutes

Cooking Time: 8 minutes

Servings: 4

Ingredients:

- 1/2 cup Fisher Sliced Almonds
- 1 cup whole milk ricotta
- 1/4 teaspoon almond extract
- zest from an orange, optional
- 1 teaspoon honey
- hearty whole-grain toast
- English muffin or bagel
- extra Fisher sliced almonds
- sliced peaches
- extra honey for drizzling

Directions:

1. Cut peaches into a proper shape and then brush them with olive oil. After that, set it aside. Take a bowl; combine the ingredients for the filling. Set aside.

2. Then just pre-heat grill to medium. Place peaches cut side down onto the greased grill. Close lid cover

and then just grill until the peaches have softened, approximately 6-10 minutes, depending on the size of the peaches.

3. Then you will have to place peach halves onto a serving plate. Put a spoon of about 1 tablespoon of ricotta mixture into the cavity (you are also allowed to use a small scooper).

4. Sprinkle it with slivered almonds, crushed amaretti cookies, and honey. Decorate with the mint leaves.

Nutrition:

Calories: 187

Protein: 7 g

Fat: 9 g

Carbs: 18 g

Mediterranean Eggs Cups

Preparation Time: 10 minutes

Cooking Time: 20 minutes

Servings: 8

Ingredients:

- 1 cup spinach, finely diced
- 1/2 yellow onion, finely diced
- 1/2 cup sliced sun-dried tomatoes
- 4 large basil leaves, finely diced
- Pepper and salt to taste
- 1/3 cup feta cheese crumbles
- 8 large eggs
- 1/4 cup milk (any kind)

Directions:

1. Warm the oven to 375°F. Then, roll the dough sheet into a 12x8-inch rectangle. Then, cut in half lengthwise.

2. After that, you will have to cut each half crosswise into 4 pieces, forming 8 (4x3-inch) pieces dough. Then, press each into the bottom and up sides of the ungreased muffin cup.

3. Trim dough to keep the dough from touching, if essential. Set aside. Then, you will have to combine

the eggs, salt, pepper in the bowl and beat it with a whisk until well mixed. Set aside.

4. Melt the butter in 12-inch skillet over medium heat until sizzling; add bell peppers. You will have to cook it, stirring occasionally, 2-3 minutes or until crisply tender.

5. After that, add spinach leaves; continue cooking until spinach is wilted. Then just add egg mixture and prosciutto.

6. Divide the mixture evenly among prepared muffin cups. Finally, bake it for 14-17 minutes or until the crust is golden brown.

Nutrition:

Calories: 240; Protein: 9 g; Fat: 16 g; Carbs: 13 g

Lunch

Caprese Pasta Salad

Preparation Time: 10 minutes

Cooking Time: 10 minutes

Servings: 6

Ingredients:

- 15 oz brown rice pasta
- 1 tbsp fresh lemon juice
- 1 tbsp garlic, minced
- 2 tbsp olive oil
- ¼ cup balsamic vinegar
- 1 avocado, chopped
- 1 cup fresh basil, chopped
- 8 oz cherry tomatoes, halved
- ¼ tsp pepper
- ½ tsp salt

Directions:

1. In a small bowl, mix together lemon juice, garlic, oil, vinegar, pepper, and salt and set aside. Cook pasta according to the packet instructions. Drain well and place in a large mixing bowl.

2. Add remaining ingredients to the bowl and mix well. Pour dressing over salad and toss well. Serve and enjoy.

Nutrition:

Calories: 378

Fat: 12.9g

Protein: 6.7g

Carbs: 59.6g

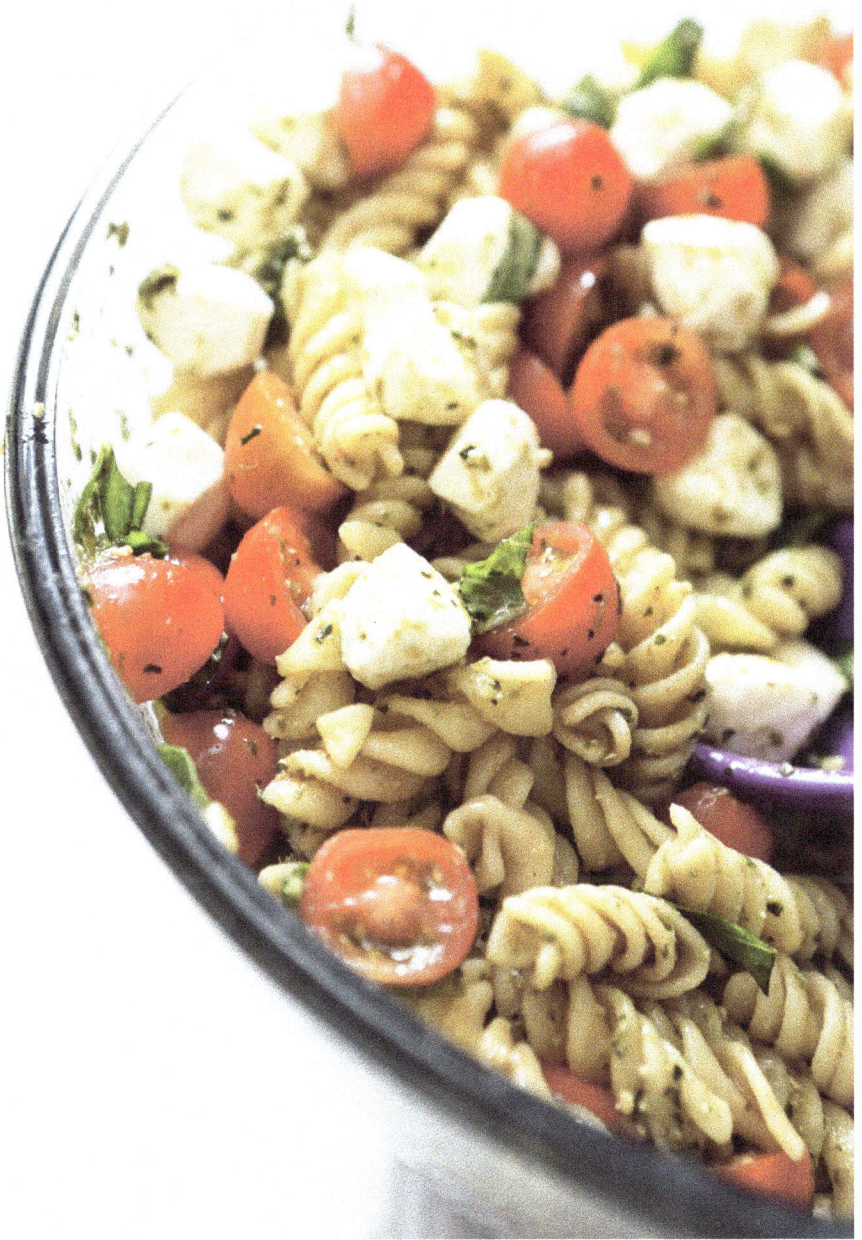

Spinach Bean Soup

Preparation Time: 10 minutes

Cooking Time: 6 hours

Servings: 6

Ingredients:

- 8 cups fresh spinach, chopped
- 1 tsp dried basil, crushed
- 1 tsp garlic, minced
- ½ cup onion, chopped
- ½ cup of brown rice
- 14.5 oz can Great Northern beans, rinsed and drained
- 14.5 oz can tomato puree
- 5 ½ cups vegetable broth
- ¼ tsp pepper
- ¼ tsp salt

Directions:

1. Add all ingredients except spinach into the slow cooker and stir well. Cover slow cooker with lid and cook on low for 6 hours. Add spinach and stir well. Serve and enjoy.

Nutrition:

Calories: 186; Fat: 2.5g; Protein: 11.8g; Carbs: 30.2g

Roasted Zucchini

Preparation Time: 10 minutes

Cooking Time: 15 minutes

Servings: 4

Ingredients:

- 1 lb. zucchini, sliced
- 1 oz parmesan cheese, grated
- 1 tsp dried mix herbs
- 1 garlic clove, minced
- 2 tbsp olive oil

Directions:

1. Preheat the oven to 450 F/ 232 C. Add all ingredients except parmesan cheese into the large bowl and toss well.
2. Transfer the zucchini mixture to the baking dish and cook in preheated oven for 10 minutes. Sprinkle parmesan cheese over zucchini. Return to the oven and cook for 5 minutes more. Serve and enjoy.

Nutrition:

Calories: 102

Fat: 8.7g

Protein: 3.7g

Carbs: 4.3g

Lemon Artichoke Salad

Preparation Time: 10 minutes

Cooking Time: 10 minutes

Servings: 4

Ingredients:

- 28 oz can artichoke hearts, drained and quartered
- 2 tbsp olive oil
- ¼ cup fresh parsley, chopped
- 2 garlic cloves, minced
- 1 lemon, chopped
- 10 oz can mushroom, drained and sliced
- Pepper
- Salt

Directions:

1. Add all ingredients into the mixing bowl and toss well. Serve immediately and enjoy.

Nutrition:

Calories: 141

Fat: 7g

Protein: 5.2g

Carbs: 14.1g

Mushroom Bean Gumbo

Preparation Time: 10 minutes

Cooking Time: 8 minutes

Servings: 4

Ingredients:

- 1 cup mushrooms, sliced
- 2 cups vegetable stock
- 2 medium zucchinis, sliced
- 2 tbsp olive oil
- 1 cup red beans, soaked overnight
- 2 garlic cloves, chopped
- 1 green bell pepper, chopped

Directions:

1. Add all ingredients into the Pressure Pot and stir well. Seal the Pressure Pot with a lid and cook on high pressure for 8 minutes.
2. Once done, allow to release pressure naturally for 10 minutes then release remaining pressure using a quick release method. Stir well and serve.

Nutrition:

Calories: 251

Fat: 8.8g

Protein: 12.5g

Carbs: 35.8g

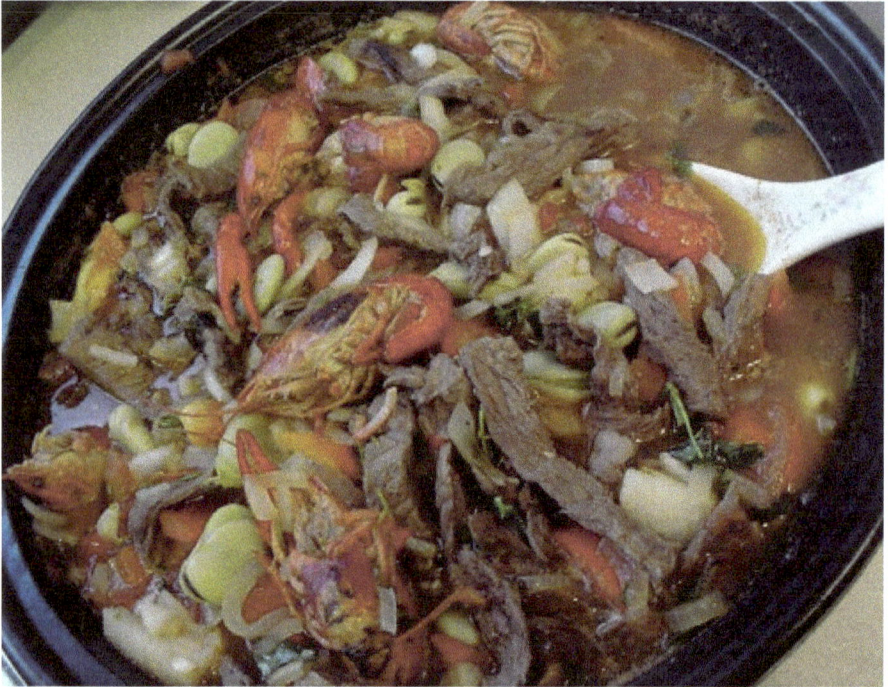

Easy Balsamic Parsnips

Preparation Time: 10 minutes

Cooking Time: 3 minutes

Servings: 4

Ingredients:

- 1 1/2 lb. parsnips, peeled and sliced
- 1/4 cup vegetable stock
- 1 tbsp honey
- 3 tbsp balsamic vinegar
- 1/8 tsp pepper
- 1/2 tsp salt

Directions:

1. Add parsnips, vinegar, and stock into the Pressure Pot. Seal pot with lid and cook on high pressure for 3 minutes.
2. Once done, release pressure using the quick release method. Open the lid. Stir in honey and season with pepper and salt. Serve and enjoy.

Nutrition:

Calories: 149

Fat: 1g

Protein: 2.1g

Carbs: 35.6g

Creamy Carrot Soup

Preparation Time: 10 minutes

Cooking Time: 45 minutes

Servings: 6

Ingredients:

- 2 lb. carrots, peeled and sliced
- 4 garlic cloves, chopped
- 2 leeks, sliced
- 2 tbsp olive oil
- 4 cups vegetable stock
- 1/2 tsp ground cumin
- 1/4 tsp ground coriander
- Pepper
- Salt

Directions:

1. Heat olive oil in a saucepan over medium heat. Add carrots, cumin, coriander, garlic, leek, pepper, and salt and cook for 15 minutes. Add stock and stir well. Bring to boil.

2. Turn heat to low and simmer for 30 minutes. Puree the soup using an immersion blender until smooth. Serve and enjoy.

Nutrition:

Calories: 125; Fat: 5.1g; Protein: 1.9g; Carbs: 20.2g

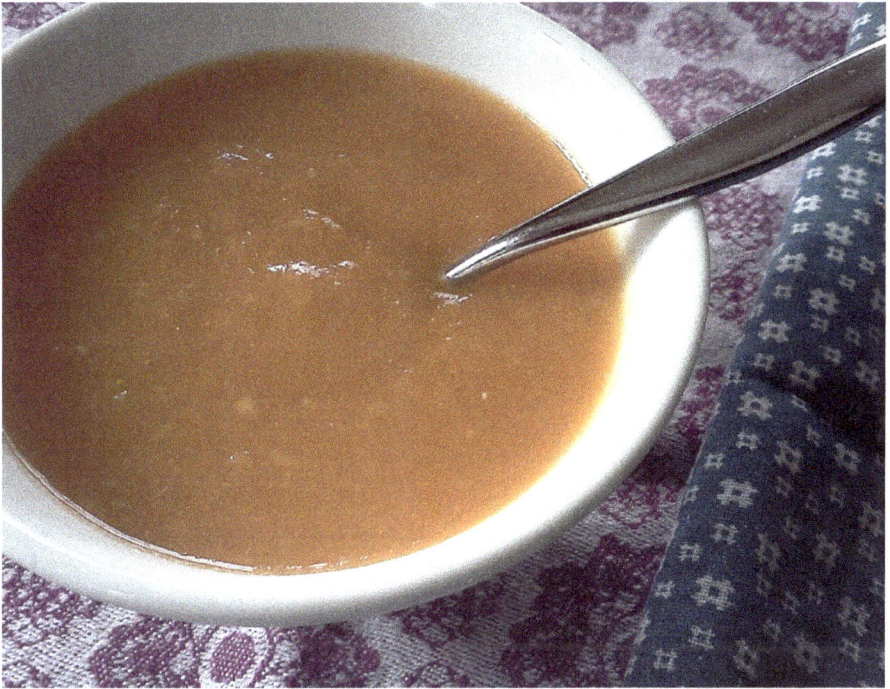

Mushroom Spinach Frittata

Preparation Time: 10 minutes

Cooking Time: 17 minutes

Servings: 6

Ingredients:

- 8 eggs
- 1/4 cup onion, diced
- 1 1/2 cup mushrooms, sliced
- 1 tbsp olive oil
- 2 cups spinach, chopped
- 1 tbsp Italian seasoning, crushed
- Pepper
- Salt

Directions:

1. Preheat the oven to 350 F/ 180 C. Heat oil in the oven-safe pan over medium-high heat. Add onion and mushrooms and sauté for 5 minutes. Add spinach and cook for 2 minutes.
2. In a large bowl, whisk eggs with Italian seasoning, pepper, and salt. Transfer pan mixture to the egg mixture and stir well.
3. Return egg mixture into the oven-safe pan and cook in preheated oven for 10 minutes. Serve and enjoy.

Nutrition:

Calories: 119; Fat: 9g; Protein: 8.3g; Carbs: 2.1g

Lemon Orzo Salad

Preparation Time: 10 minutes

Cooking Time: 15 minutes

Servings: 6

Ingredients:

- 12 oz whole wheat orzo pasta
- ¼ cup olive oil
- 1 lemon juice
- 1 cup fresh mint leaves, chopped
- 1 cup fresh basil leaves, chopped
- ½ small onion, diced
- 1 cucumber, diced
- 14.5 oz can chickpeas, rinsed and drained
- 3 cups baby spinach, chopped
- Pepper
- Salt

Directions:

1. Cook pasta according to the packet instructions. Drain well and place in a large mixing bowl. Add remaining ingredients to the bowl and toss well.
2. Season salad with pepper and salt. Serve and enjoy.

Nutrition:

Calories: 381; Fat: 10.6g; Protein: 11.7g; Carbs: 65.3g

Avocado Tomato Salad

Preparation Time: 10 minutes

Cooking Time: 5 minutes

Servings: 4

Ingredients:

- 2 avocados, diced
- ½ onion, diced
- 1 tbsp olive oil
- ¼ cup fresh cilantro, chopped
- 1 fresh lime juice
- 4 cups cherry tomatoes, halved
- Pepper
- Salt

Directions:

1. Add all ingredients into the mixing bowl and toss well. Serve and enjoy.

Nutrition:

Calories: 276

Fat: 23.5g

Protein: 3.7g

Carbs: 17.9

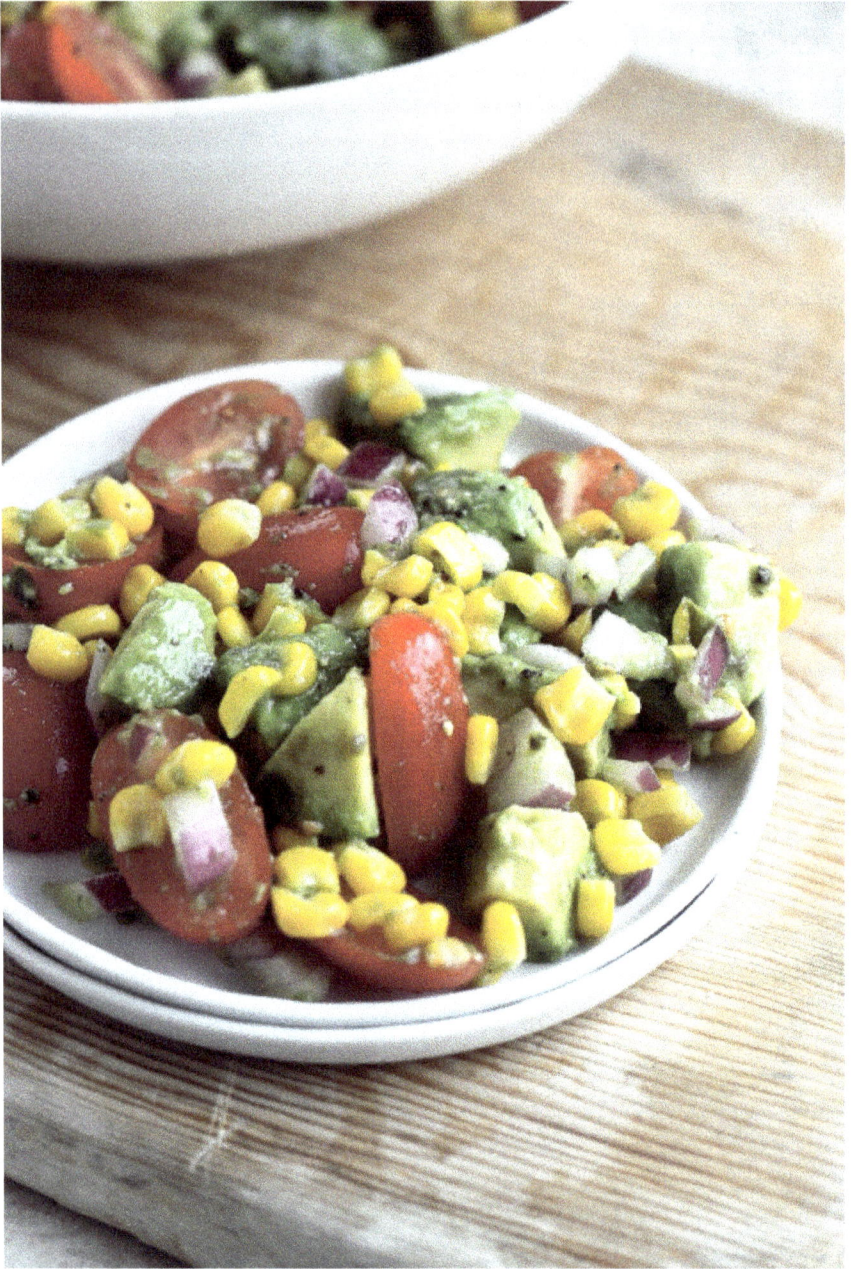

Creamy Corn

Preparation Time: 10 minutes

Cooking Time: 20 minutes

Servings: 4

Ingredients:

- 2 cups corn
- 2 cups cherry tomatoes, halved
- 1 cup coconut milk
- 1 tablespoon mint, chopped
- 1 teaspoon turmeric powder
- 1 teaspoon chili powder
- A pinch of salt and black pepper
- 2 tablespoons green onions, chopped

Directions:

1. In a pan, combine the corn with the cherry tomatoes, the milk and the other ingredients, toss, bring to a simmer and cook over medium heat for 20 minutes.
2. Divide the mix between plates and serve as a side dish.

Nutrition:

Calories 199

Fat 2

Fiber 3

Carbs 8

Protein 6

Balsamic Squash Mix

Preparation Time: 10 minutes

Cooking Time: 25 minutes

Servings: 4

Ingredients:

- 1 butternut squash, peeled and roughly cubed
- 2 spring onions, chopped
- 1 tablespoon avocado oil
- A pinch of salt and black pepper
- 1 tablespoon balsamic vinegar
- 1 tablespoon cilantro, chopped
- 1/2 cup pecans, toasted and chopped

Directions:

1. In a roasting pan, combine the squash with the spring onions and the other ingredients, toss and bake.
2. Divide the mix between plates and serve.

Nutrition:

Calories 211

Fat 3

Fiber 4

Carbs 9

Protein 6

Cinnamon and Ginger Carrots Mix

Preparation Time: 10 minutes

Cooking Time: 30 minutes

Servings: 2

Ingredients:

- 1 pound baby carrots, peeled
- 1 tablespoon ginger, grated
- 3 tablespoons cinnamon powder
- 1 tablespoon coconut oil, melted
- 1 tablespoon chives, chopped

Directions:

1. Scatter the carrots on a baking sheet lined with parchment paper, add the ginger and the other ingredients, toss and bake at 380 degrees F for 30 minutes.
2. Divide everything between plates and serve.

Nutrition:

Calories 198

Fat 2

Fiber 4

Carbs 11

Protein 6

Rice and Tomato Salad

Preparation Time: 10 minutes

Cooking Time: 0 minutes

Servings: 4

Ingredients:

- 2 tablespoons olive oil
- 2 cups brown rice, cooked
- 1/2 cup cherry tomatoes, halved
- 2 teaspoons cumin, ground
- 1/4 cup cilantro, chopped
- A pinch of salt and black pepper
- 2 tablespoons olive oil

Directions:

1. In a bowl, combine the rice with the oil and the other ingredients, toss and serve.

Nutrition:

Calories 122

Fat 4

Fiber 3

Carbs 8

Protein 5

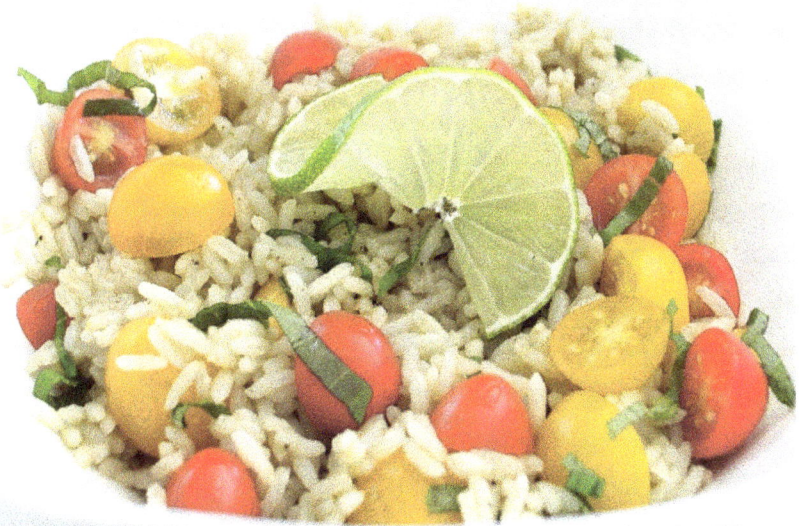

Dinner

Chicken Cacciatore

Preparation Time: 10 minutes

Cooking Time: 6-8 Hours

Servings: 4

Ingredients

- 1/4 teaspoon of pepper and salt
- 1/4 cup of fresh basil
- 1 large zucchini (12 ounces
- 1 bay leaf
- Diced tomatoes
- 1 (15 ounces) can of petite
- 1 cup of button mushrooms, should be halved
- 1 small bell pepper, with the seeds and membranes removed
- 2 scallions, should be minced
- 2 cloves of garlic, should be minced
- 4 (7 ounces) raw bone-in, skinless chicken thighs (1 3/4 pound in total).

Directions:

1. Combine pepper, salt, bay leaf, tomatoes, mushrooms, bell peppers, garlic, and chicken in a slow cooker and set to low for 6-8 hours

2. Before you serve, whisk in the basil and zucchini noodles. Then mix thoroughly to combine.

Nutrition:

Calories310

Protein38g

Carbohydrate15g

Fat 2 G

Crock Pot Chicken Taco Soup

Preparation Time: 10 minutes

Cooking Time: 4 hours

Servings: 4

Ingredients

- 2 oz. Cheese for garnishing
- 2 cups of cabbage, chopped
- 13-14 oz. of raw chicken breasts
- 1 clove of garlic, should be minced
- 1/4 teaspoon of chili powder
- 1/2 teaspoon of cumin
- 1 teaspoon of reduced-sodium taco seasoning mix
- 1 cup of Rotel diced tomatoes with green chilies
- 2 cups of water
- 2 cups of reduced-sodium chicken broth

Directions:

1. Combine chicken, cabbage, garlic, chili powder, cumin, taco seasoning, diced tomatoes, water, and chicken broth in a crockpot.
2. Cook under high heat for 3-4 hours or under low heat for 6-8 hours.
3. It would be best if you shredded the chicken breast inside the crockpot before you serve.

4. Finally, pour the soup inside the bowls before topping with cheese.

Nutrition:

Calories: 338

Protein: 28g

Total Carbohydrates: 16g

Sugars: 10g

Saturated Fat: 4g

Crock Pot Chili

Preparation Time: 10 minutes

Cooking Time: 8 Hours

Servings: 5

Ingredients:

- 1 teaspoon of stevia
- 3/4 teaspoon of salt
- 1/2 teaspoon of black pepper
- 1 teaspoon of cumin
- 1 1/2 tablespoon of chili powder
- 1/2 teaspoon of garlic powder
- 1/2 cup of green peppers, should be diced
- 1/2 cup of water
- 1/2 cup of Great Value natural tomato sauce
- 2 cans (14.5 oz. each) of Great value Italian diced tomatoes
- 25 oz. of lean cooked ground beef

Directions:

1. Combine all the ingredients inside a crockpot and cook on LOW heat for 8 hours. Once done, serve and enjoy.

Nutrition:

Calories: 379; Protein: 35g; Total Carbohydrates: 10g; Total Fat: 20g ; Saturated Fat: 4g

Easy Turkey Chili

Preparation Time: 10 minutes

Cooking Time: 40 Minutes

Servings: 4

Ingredients

- 1/4 teaspoon of salt
- 1/4 teaspoon red pepper flakes
- 2 teaspoon of chili powder
- 1 1/2 teaspoon of ground cumin
- 1 cup of water (optional)
- 1, 28 ounces can of diced tomatoes
- 2 teaspoons of olive oil
- 1 jalapeno pepper, should be diced
- 1 medium green bell pepper, should be diced
- 1 medium red bell pepper, should be diced
- 2 garlic cloves, should be minced
- 2 tablespoon of diced onion
- 1 1/2 lb. 99% lean ground turkey
- Toppings (Per Serving)
- 3 tablespoon of low-fat shredded cheddar cheese
- 2 tablespoon of low-fat plain Greek Yogurt
- 2oz. of avocado, diced
- 2 tablespoons of chopped scallions

Directions:

1. Put a large soup pot on medium-high heat and sauté peppers, garlic, and onions in oil for about 4-5 minutes or till they become tender. Next is to add turkey and cook until it becomes brown with no traces of pink color.
2. Pour in the salt, red pepper flakes, chili powder, cumin, water (optional), and tomatoes and mix very well until they blend. Cover on low heat for 20 minutes. Serve with the toppings.

Nutrition:

Calories 464 Fat 15.3 g Carbohydrates 48.9 g Sugar 2.8 g Protein 32.2 g

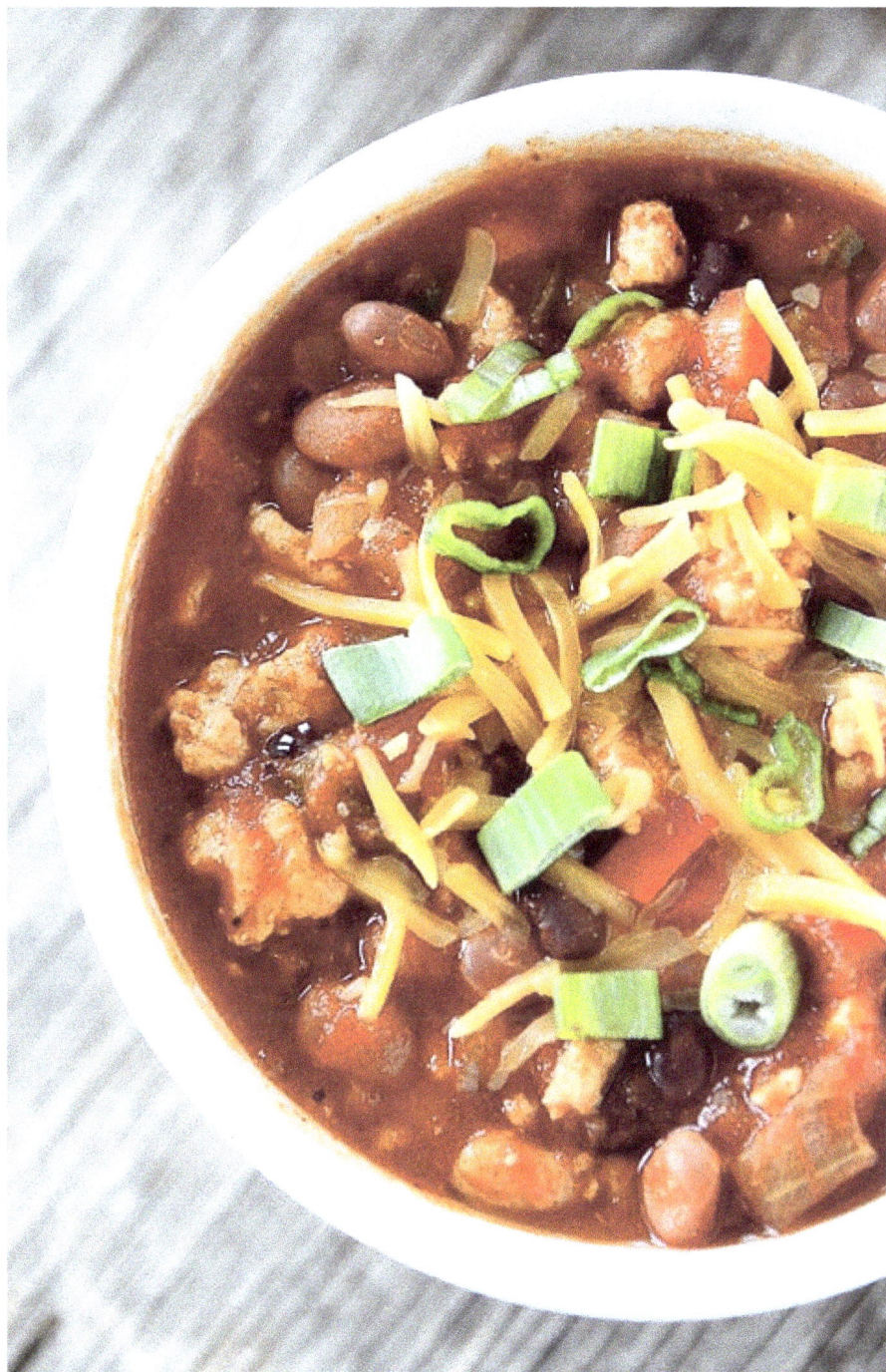

Chard and Spring Onions Mix

Preparation Time: 10 minutes

Cooking Time: 15 minutes

Servings: 4

Ingredients:

- 2 spring onions, chopped
- 4 cups red chard, shredded
- 2 tablespoons olive oil
- 2 teaspoons ginger, grated
- 1/2 teaspoon red pepper flakes, crushed
- 2 tablespoons balsamic vinegar
- 1 tablespoon chives,

Directions:

1. Heat the oil in a pan, attach the spring onions and the ginger and sauté for 5 minutes.
2. Add the chard and the other ingredients, toss, cook for 10 minutes more, divide between plates and serve as a side dish.

Nutrition:

Calories 160

Fat 10

Fiber 3

Carbs 10

Protein 5

Cabbage and Walnuts Mix

Preparation Time: 10 minutes

Cooking Time: 0 minutes

Servings: 4

Ingredients:

- 1 cup green cabbage, shredded
- 1 cup tomatoes, cubed
- 2 tablespoons walnuts, chopped
- 1 bunch green onions, chopped
- 1/4 cup balsamic vinegar
- 2 tablespoons olive oil
- 1 tablespoon chives, chopped
- A pinch of salt and black pepper

Directions:

1. In a salad bowl, mix the cabbage with the tomatoes, the walnuts and the other ingredients, toss and serve as a side dish.

Nutrition:

Calories 140

Fat 3

Fiber 3

Carbs 8

Protein 6

Balsamic Carrots and Scallions Salad

Preparation Time: 10 minutes

Cooking Time: 0 minutes

Servings: 4

Ingredients:

- 3 scallions, chopped
- 1 pound carrots, peeled and sliced
- 1/2 cup cilantro, chopped
- 3 tablespoons sesame seeds
- 2 tablespoons balsamic vinegar
- 2 tablespoons olive oil
- A pinch of salt and black pepper

Directions:

1. In a salad bowl, mix the carrots with the scallions and the other ingredients, toss well and serve as a side dish.

Nutrition:

Calories 140

Fat 4

Fiber 3

Carbs 5

Protein 6

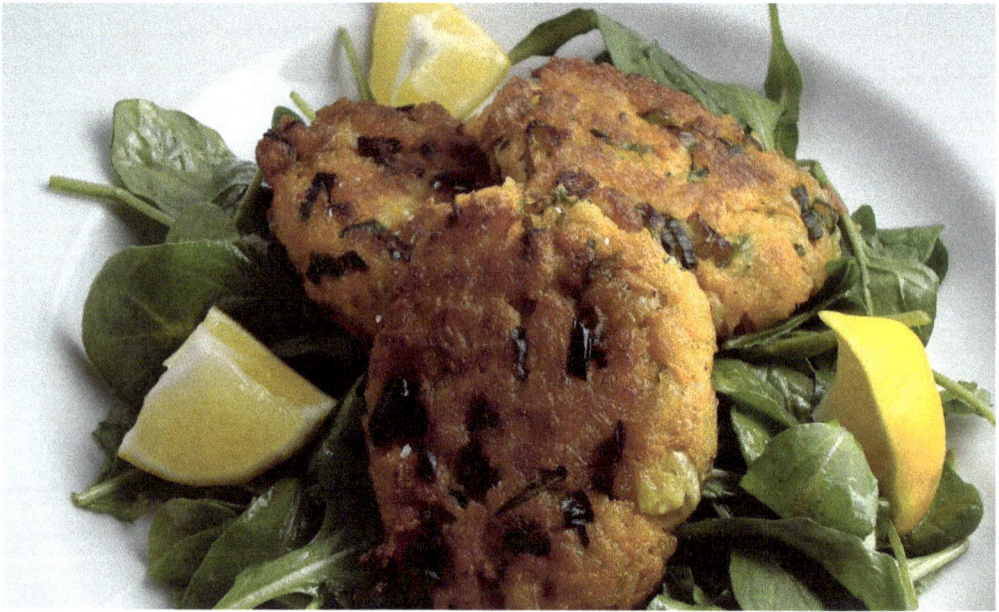

Sweet Potatoes and Walnuts Mix

Preparation Time: 1- minutes

Cooking Time: 30 minutes

Servings: 4

Ingredients:

- 2 sweet potatoes
- 2 tablespoons raisins
- 2 garlic cloves, minced
- 2 tablespoons walnuts, chopped
- Juice of 1/2 lemon
- 2 tablespoons olive oil
- A pinch of salt and black pepper

Directions:

1. In a roasting pan, combine the sweet potatoes with the raisins and the other ingredients, toss and bake at 370 degrees F.
2. Divide everything between plates and serve.

Nutrition:

Calories 120

Fat 1

Fiber 2

Carbs 3

Protein 5

Coconut Okra

Preparation Time: 10 minutes

Cooking Time: 30 minutes

Servings: 4

Ingredients:

- 2 cups okra, sliced
- 1 teaspoon turmeric powder
- A pinch of salt and black pepper
- 1 teaspoon thyme, dried
- 2 tablespoons olive oil
- 1 tablespoon coconut amino
- 1 tablespoon cilantro, chopped

Directions:

1. In a baking dish, combine the okra with the turmeric, salt, pepper and the other ingredients, toss and cook at 360 degrees F for 30 minutes.
2. Divide the mix between plates and serve as a side dish.

Nutrition:

Calories 87

Fat 7.2

Fiber 1.8

Carbs 5

Protein 1

Flank Steak with Artichokes

Preparation Time: 15 minutes

Cooking Time: 60 minutes

Servings: 4-6

Ingredients:

- 4 tablespoons grapeseed oil, divided
- 2 pounds flank steak
- 1 (14-ounce) can artichoke hearts, drained and roughly chopped
- 1 onion, diced
- 8 garlic cloves, chopped
- 1 (32-ounce) container low-sodium beef broth
- 1 (14.5-ounce) can diced tomatoes, drained
- 1 cup tomato sauce
- 2 tablespoons tomato paste
- 1 teaspoon dried oregano
- 1 teaspoon dried parsley
- 1 teaspoon dried basil
- ½ teaspoon ground cumin
- 3 bay leaves
- 2 to 3 cups cooked couscous (optional)

Directions:

1. Preheat the oven to 450ºF. In an oven-safe sauté pan or skillet, heat 3 tablespoons of oil on medium heat. Sear the steak for 2 minutes per side on both sides. Transfer the steak to the oven for 30 minutes, or until desired tenderness.

2. Meanwhile, in a large pot, combine the remaining 1 tablespoon of oil, artichoke hearts, onion, and garlic.

3. Pour in the beef broth, tomatoes, tomato sauce, and tomato paste. Stir in oregano, parsley, basil, cumin, and bay leaves.

4. Cook the vegetables, covered, for 30 minutes. Remove bay leaf and serve with flank steak and ½ cup of couscous per plate, if using.

Nutrition:

Calories: 577 ; Protein: 55g ; Carbohydrates: 22g ; Fat: 28g

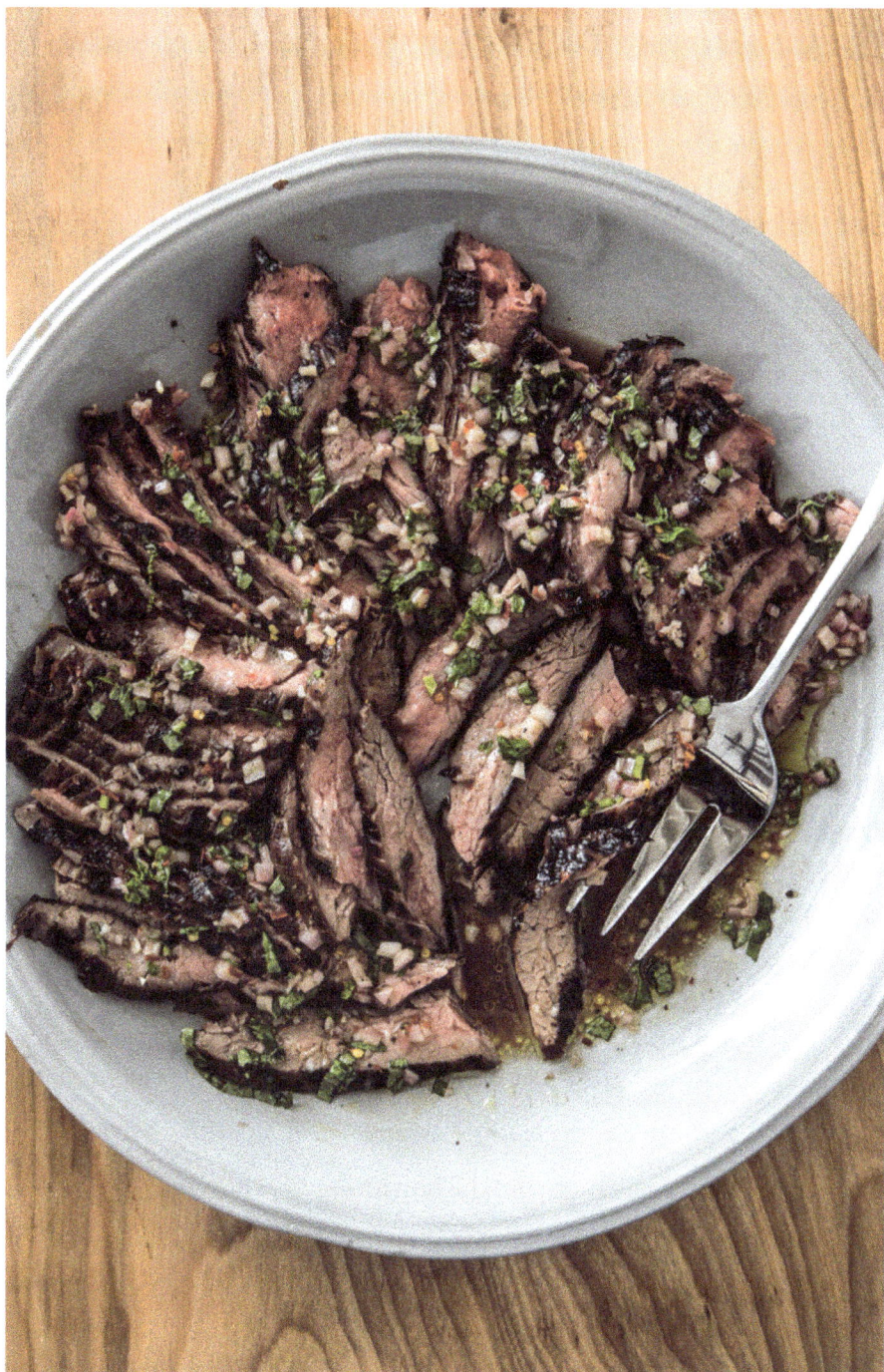

Easy Honey-Garlic Pork Chops

Preparation Time: 15 minutes

Cooking Time: 25 minutes

Servings: 4

Ingredients:

- 4 pork chops, boneless or bone-in
- ¼ teaspoon salt
- 1/8 teaspoon freshly ground black pepper
- 3 tablespoons extra-virgin olive oil
- 5 tablespoons low-sodium chicken broth, divided
- 6 garlic cloves, minced
- ¼ cup honey
- 2 tablespoons apple cider vinegar

Directions:

1. Season the pork chops with salt and pepper and set aside.
2. In a large sauté pan or skillet, heat the oil over medium-high heat. Add the pork chops and sear for 5 minutes on each side, or until golden brown.
3. Once the searing is complete, move the pork to a dish and reduce the skillet heat from medium-high to medium.

4. Add 3 tablespoons of chicken broth to the pan; this will loosen the bits and flavors from the bottom of the skillet.
5. Once the broth has evaporated, add the garlic to the skillet and cook for 15 to 20 seconds, until fragrant.
6. Add the honey, vinegar, and the remaining 2 tablespoons of broth. Bring the heat back up to medium-high and continue to cook for 3 to 4 minutes.
7. Stir periodically; the sauce is ready once it's thickened slightly. Add the pork chops back into the pan, cover them with the sauce, and cook for 2 minutes. Serve.

Nutrition:

Calories: 302; Protein: 22g; Carbohydrates: 19g ; Fat: 16g

Dessert

Coconut-Date Pudding

Preparation Time: 10 minutes, plus 3 hours to chill

Cooking Time: 10 minutes

Servings: 2

Ingredients:

- 3 cups unsweetened coconut milk, divided
- 1½ cups pitted Medrol dates, chopped
- 4 tablespoons (¼ cup) chopped walnuts
- 3 tablespoons water
- 1 teaspoon gelatin
- 1 teaspoon ground cinnamon

Directions:

1. In a medium saucepan, bring 1 cup of coconut milk and the dates to a boil. Reduce heat to medium-low, and continue cooking, stirring often, until the liquid evaporates, about 5 minutes.

2. Divide the dates between the 4 ramekins, pressing them into the bottom. Top the dates in each ramekin with 1 tablespoon of walnuts.

3. Add the remaining 2 cups of coconut milk to the saucepan, and heat over medium heat.

4. In a small bowl, whisk the water and gelatin, then add to the saucepan. Bring to a boil, reduce heat to medium, and whisk for about 5 minutes, until the gelatin is incorporated. Add the cinnamon, stirring to blend. Remove from heat and allow to slightly cool.

5. Pour the coconut mixture evenly between the 4 ramekins. Loosely cover with plastic wrap, and refrigerate the puddings to set for at least 3 hours or up to overnight.

Nutrition:

Calories: 334; Total Fat: 10g; Saturated Fat: 9g; Protein: 5g; Carbohydrates: 67g; Fiber: 8g; Sodium: 46mg

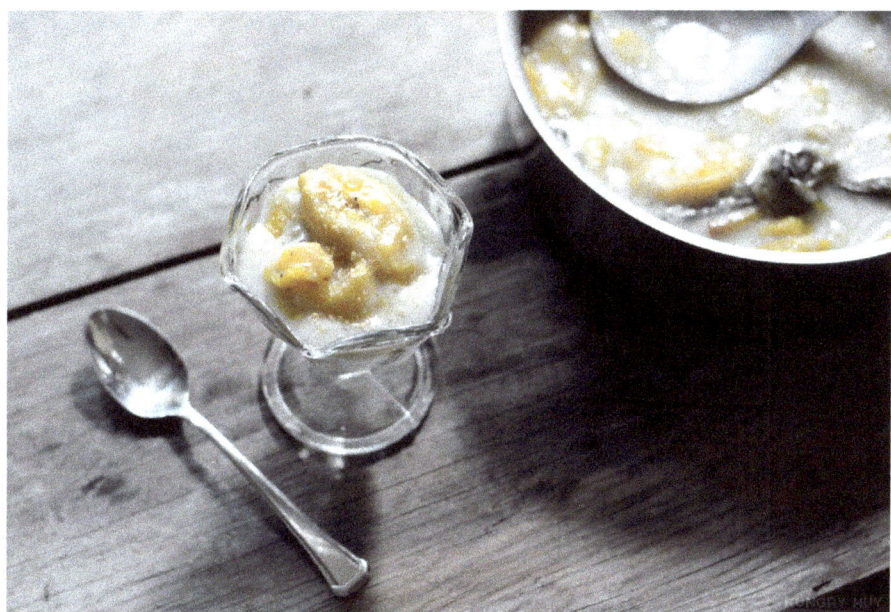

Biscuit Donuts

Preparation Time: 7 minutes

Cooking Time: 5 minutes

Servings: 8

Ingredients:

- Pinch of allspice
- tbsp. dark brown sugar
- 1 tsp. cinnamon
- 1/3cups granulated sweetener
- tbsp. melted coconut oil
- 1 can of biscuits

Directions:

1. Mix allspice, sugar, sweetener, and cinnamon.
2. Take out biscuits from can and with a circle cookie cutter, cut holes from centers, and place into the air fryer.
3. Cook 5 minutes at 350 °F
4. As batches are cooked, use a brush to coat with melted coconut oil and dip each into sugar mixture.
5. Serve warm!

Nutrition:

Calories 378; Fat9g; Carbs5g; Protein 4g

Angel Food Cake

Preparation Time: 5 minutes

Cooking Time: 30 minutes

Servings: 12

Ingredients:

- ¼ cup butter, melted
- 1 cup powdered erythritol
- 1 teaspoon strawberry extract
- 12 egg whites
- 2 teaspoons cream of tartar

Directions:

1. Preheat the air fryer oven for 5 minutes.
2. Blend the cream of tartar and egg whites.
3. Use a hand mixer and whisk until white and fluffy.
4. Add the rest of the ingredients except for the butter and whisk for another minute.
5. Pour into a baking dish.
6. Place in the air fryer basket and cook for 30 minutes at 400°F or if a toothpick inserted in the middle comes out clean.
7. Drizzle with melted butter once cooled.

Nutrition:

Calories – 65; Protein – 3.1 g; Fat – 5 g; Carbs – 6.2 g

Cream Cheese Wontons

Preparation Time: 5 minutes

Cooking Time: 5 minutes

Servings: 16

Ingredients:

- 1 egg mixed with a bit of water
- Wonton wrappers
- ½cup powdered erythritol
- oz. softened cream cheese Olive oil

Directions:

1. Mix sweetener and cream cheese together.
2. Lay out four wontons at a time and cover with a dish towel to prevent drying out.
3. Place ½ of a tsp. of cream cheese mixture into each wrapper
4. Dip finger into egg/water mixture and fold diagonally to form a triangle.
5. Seal edges well and repeat the same with the remaining ingredients.
6. Place filled wontons into the Smart Air Fryer Oven and cook 5 minutes at 400 °F, shaking halfway through cooking.

Nutrition:

Calories 378

Fat9g

Carbs5g

Protein 4g

Cinnamon Rolls

Preparation Time: 2 hours 11 minutes

Cooking Time: 5 minutes

Servings: 8

Ingredients:

- 1 ½ tbsp. cinnamon
- ¾ cups brown sugar
- ¼ cups melted coconut oil
- 1 lb. frozen bread dough, thawed

Glaze:

- ½ tsp. vanilla
- 1 ¼ cups powdered erythritol
- tbsp. softened ghee
- oz. softened cream cheese

Directions:

1. Lay out bread dough and roll out into a rectangle.
2. Brush melted ghee over the dough and leave a 1-inch border along edges.
3. Mix cinnamon and sweetener and then sprinkle over dough.
4. Roll dough tightly and slice into 8 pieces.
5. Let sit for 2 hours to rise

6. To make the glaze, simply mix the glaze ingredients till smooth.

7. Once rolls rise, place into the air fryer and cook 5 minutes at 350 °F.

8. Serve rolls drizzled in cream cheese glaze.

9. Enjoy!

Nutrition:

Calories 378, Fat9g, Carbs5g, Protein 4g

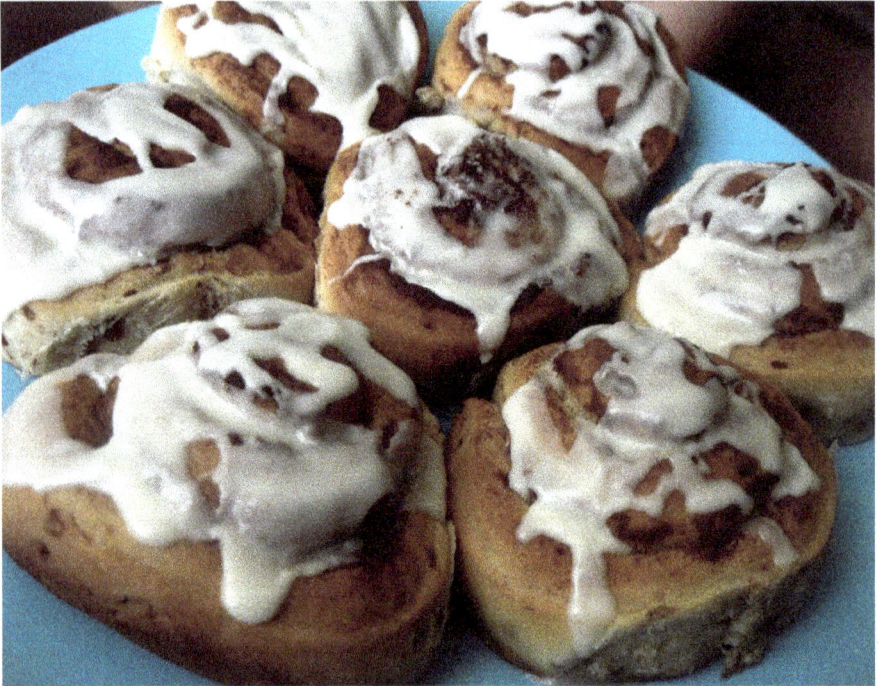

Honey Fruit Compote

Preparation Time: 10 minutes

Cooking Time: 3 minutes

Servings: 4

Ingredients:

- 1/3 cup honey
- 1 1/2 cups blueberries
- 1 1/2 cups raspberries

Directions:

1. Put all of the ingredients in the air fryer basket and stir well.
2. Seal pot with lid and cook on high for 3 minutes.
3. Once done, allow to release pressure naturally. Remove lid.
4. Serve and enjoy.

Nutrition:

Calories – 141

Protein – 1 g.

Fat – 0.5 g.

Carbs – 36.7 g.

Yogurt Mint

Preparation Time: 5 minutes

Cooking Time: 10 minutes

Servings: 2

Ingredients:

- 1 cup of water
- 5 cups of milk
- 3/4 cup plain yogurt
- 1/4 cup fresh mint
- 1 tbsp. maple syrup

Directions:

1. Attach 1 cup water to the Pressure Pot Pressure Cooker.
2. Press the STEAM function button and adjust to 1 minute.
3. Once done, add the milk, then press the YOGURT function button and allow boiling.
4. Add yogurt and fresh mint, then stir well.
5. Pour into a glass and add maple syrup.
6. Enjoy.

Nutrition:

Calories: 25; Fat: 0.5 g; Carbs: 5 g; Protein: 2 g

Chocolate Fondue

Preparation Time: 5 minutes

Cooking Time: 10 minutes

Servings: 2

Ingredients:

- 1 cup water
- 1/2 tsp. sugar
- 1/2 cup coconut cream
- 3/4 cup dark chocolate, chopped

Directions:

1. Pour the water into your Pressure Pot.
2. To a heatproof bowl, add the chocolate, sugar, and coconut cream.
3. Place in the Pressure Pot.
4. Seal the lid, select MANUAL, and cook for 2 minutes. When ready, do a quick release and carefully open the lid. Stir well and serve immediately.

Nutrition:

Calories: 216

Fat: 17 g

Carbs: 11 g

Protein: 2 g

Rice Pudding

Preparation Time: 5 minutes

Cooking Time: 12 minutes

Servings: 2

Ingredients:

- 1/2 cup short grain rice
- 1/4 cup of sugar
- 1 cinnamon stick
- 11/2 cup milk
- 1 slice lemon peel
- Salt to taste

Directions:

1. Rinse the rice under cold water.
2. Put the milk, cinnamon stick, sugar, salt, and lemon peel inside the Pressure Pot Pressure Cooker.
3. Close the lid, lock in place, and make sure to seal the valve. Press the PRESSURE button and cook for 10 minutes on HIGH.
4. When the timer beeps, choose the QUICK PRESSURE release. This will take about 2 minutes.
5. Remove the lid. Open the pressure cooker and discard the lemon peel and cinnamon stick. Spoon in a serving bowl and serve.

Nutrition:

Calories: 111; Fat: 6 g; Carbs: 21 g; Protein: 3 g

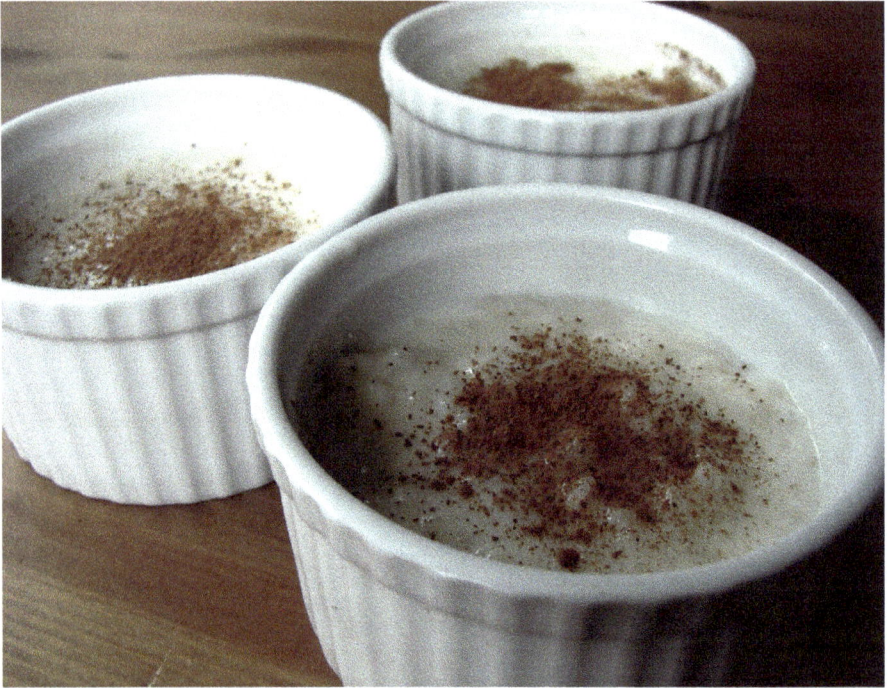

Braised Apples

Preparation Time: 5 minutes

Cooking Time: 12 minutes

Servings: 2

Ingredients:

- 2 cored apples
- 1/2 cup of water
- 1/2 cup red wine
- 3 tbsp. sugar
- 1/2 tsp. ground cinnamon

Directions:

1. In the bottom of Pressure Pot, add the water and place apples.
2. Pour wine on top and sprinkle with sugar and cinnamon. Close the lid carefully and cook for 10 minutes at HIGH PRESSURE.
3. When done, do a quick pressure release.
4. Transfer the apples onto serving plates and top with cooking liquid.
5. Serve immediately.

Nutrition:

Calories: 24; Fat: 0.5 g; Carbs: 53 g; Protein: 1 g

Wine Figs

Preparation Time: 5 minutes

Cooking Time: 3 minutes

Servings: 2

Ingredients:

- 1/2 cup pine nuts
- 1 cup red wine
- 1 lb. figs
- Sugar, as needed

Directions:

1. Slowly pour the wine and sugar into the Pressure Pot.
2. Arrange the trivet inside it; place the figs over it. Close the lid and lock. Ensure that you have sealed the valve to avoid leakage.
3. Press MANUAL mode and set timer to 3 minutes.
4. After the timer reads zero, press CANCEL and quick-release pressure.
5. Carefully remove the lid.
6. Divide figs into bowls, and drizzle wine from the pot over them.
7. Top with pine nuts and enjoy.

Nutrition:

Calories: 9; Fat: 3 g; Carbs: 5 g; Protein: 2 g

Cinnamon Chickpeas Cookies

Preparation Time: 10 minutes

Cooking Time: 20 minutes

Servings: 12

Ingredients:

- 1 cup canned chickpeas
- 2 cups almond flour
- 1 teaspoon cinnamon powder
- 1 teaspoon baking powder
- 1 cup avocado oil
- 1/2 cup stevia
- 1 egg, whisked
- 2 teaspoons almond extract
- 1 cup raisins
- 1 cup coconut, unsweetened and shredded

Directions:

1. In a bowl, combine the chickpeas with the flour, cinnamon and the other ingredients, and whisk well until you obtain a dough.
2. Scoop tablespoons of dough on a baking sheet lined with parchment paper, introduce in oven for 20 minutes at 350 degrees. Let it cool and serve.

Nutrition:

Calories 200; Fat 4.5g; Carbohydrates 9.5g; Protein 2.4g

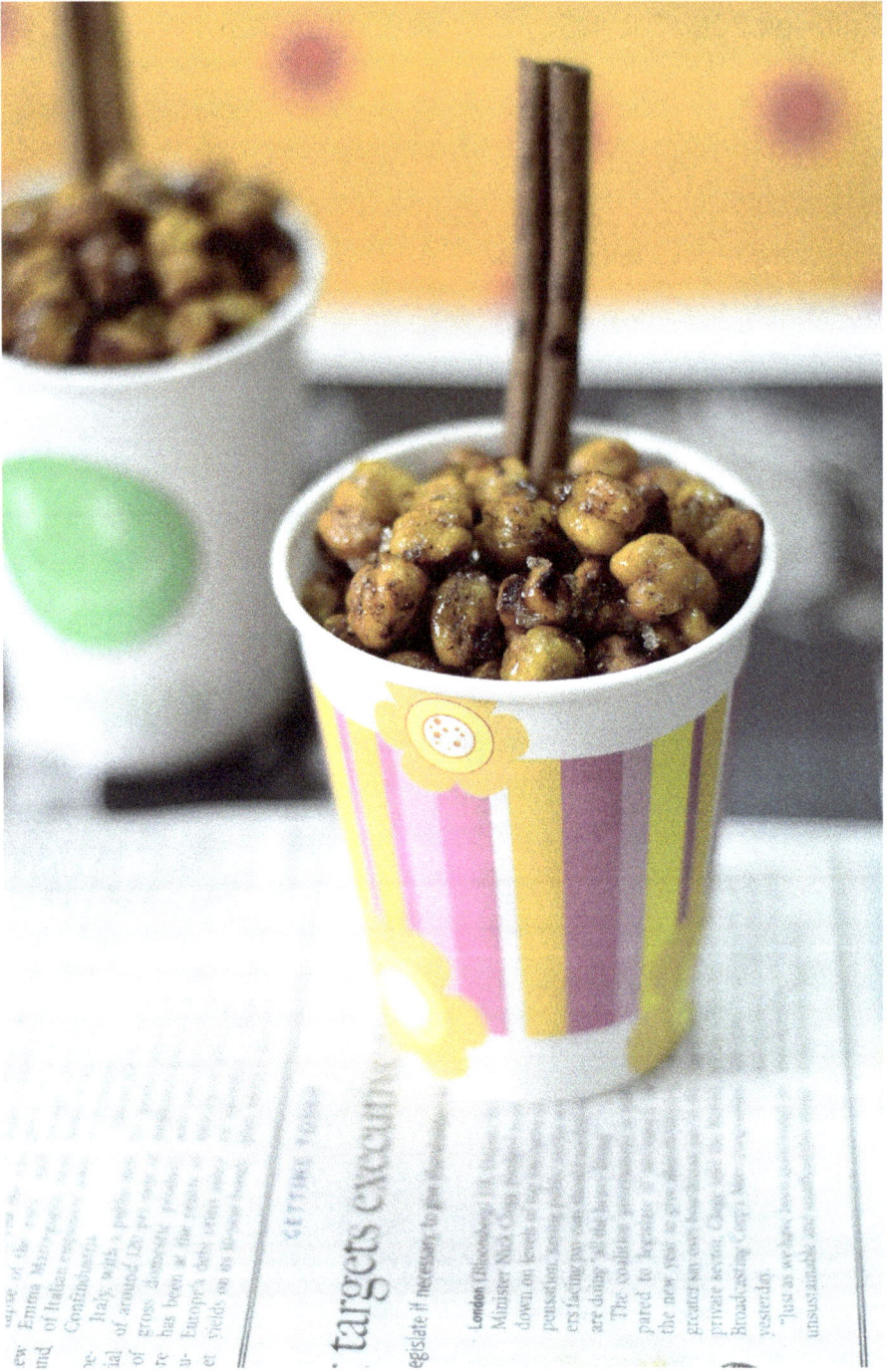

www.ingramcontent.com/pod-product-compliance
Lightning Source LLC
Chambersburg PA
CBHW050755030426
42336CB00012B/1827